THE *Skinny*
FRUIT-INFUSED
WATER
RECIPE BOOK

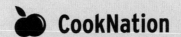

CookNation

THE SKINNY FRUIT-INFUSED WATER RECIPE BOOK
DELICIOUS, DETOXING, NO-CALORIE VITAMIN WATER TO HELP BOOST YOUR METABOLISM, LOSE WEIGHT AND FEEL GREAT!

ISBN 978-1-910771-42-6

A CIP catalogue record of this book is available from the British Library

DISCLAIMER

This book is designed to provide information on fruit-infused water drinks that can be made using fruit-infuser bottles and pitchers, results may differ if alternative devices are used.

Some recipes may contain nuts or traces of nuts. Those suffering from any allergies associated with nuts should avoid any recipes containing nuts or nut based oils.

This information is provided and sold with the knowledge that the publisher and author do not offer any legal or other professional advice.

In the case of a need for any such expertise consult with the appropriate professional.

This book does not contain all information available on the subject, and other sources of recipes are available.

This book has not been created to be specific to any individual's requirements.

Every effort has been made to make this book as accurate as possible. However, there may be typographical and or content errors. Therefore, this book should serve only as a general guide and not as the ultimate source of subject information.

This book contains information that might be dated and is intended only to educate and entertain.

The author and publisher shall have no liability or responsibility to any person or entity regarding any loss or damage incurred, or alleged to have incurred, directly or indirectly, by the information contained in this book.

CONTENTS

INTRODUCTION

OTHER COOKNATION TITLES

INTRODUCTION

Whether you are looking to lose weight, detox your body of just enjoy great tasting refreshing drinks then fruit infused water is for you.

All our fruit infused water recipes are simple, quick and easy: generally a combination of fresh fruits, vegetables, and herbs immersed in cold water although you can use frozen fruit where appropriate and some of the recipes suggest sparkling water.

All the recipe ideas in this book have been developed for use in a 750ml/3 cup size fruit infuser sports bottle but you can easily alter the quantities to make a single glass or large pitcher jug which you can leave cooling in the fridge and go back to time and time again.

Experts suggest that the average person should consume at least 1.75lt/7 cups of water per day, boosting your metabolism, flushing toxins from your system, improving your mood and because infused waters are naturally low in calories and contain no artificial ingredients, you can drink as much of it as you want. So if it's weight loss you are looking to achieve you will find drinking fruit-infused water will aid your dieting efforts by filling you up and suppressing your hunger pangs.

All of the recipes in this book are suggestions, but there's no reason why you can't have fun creating your own drinks using some of the basic ingredients which you will find mentioned time and again in some of the most popular fruit infused water recipes.

Some of the most common ingredients are:

Lemons

The health benefits of lemons come from its numerous vitamins and minerals including: vitamin C, vitamin B6, vitamin A, vitamin E, folate, niacin thiamin, riboflavin, pantothenic acid, copper, calcium, iron, magnesium, potassium, zinc, phosphorus and protein.

They contains vital flavonoids, which are composites that contain antioxidant and cancer fighting properties. It helps to prevent diabetes, constipation, high blood pressure, fever, indigestion and many other problems, as well as improving the skin, hair, and teeth.

Oranges

Oranges are an excellent source of Vitamin C as well as being packed with dietary fibre, B vitamins, calcium, copper, and potassium.

Apples

Often referred to as nutritional powerhouses. Apples contain Vitamin C, riboflavin, thiamin, vitamin B-6, dietary fibre, calcium, potassium & phosphorus.

Strawberries

Strawberries are a wonderful source of vitamins C and K as well as providing a good dose of fibre, folic acid, manganese & potassium. In addition their fibre and fructose content is thought the help regulate blood sugar levels by slowing digestion.

Watermelon

Watermelons are a refreshing fruit made up of over 90% water which is soaked with nutrients including vitamins A, B6 and C as well as lycopene, antioxidants & amino acids.

Mint

Mint has one of the highest antioxidant capacities of any food. One of its properties rosmarinic acid is thought to be effective in relieving seasonal allergy symptoms.

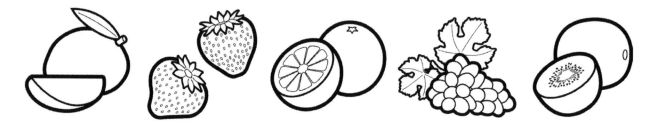

Mango

Hailed as the 'king' of fruits. Studies suggest mangos may help to alkalize the body, aid weight loss, regulate diabetes, help digestion & cleanse your skin.

Cinnamon

For hundreds of years cinnamon has been used as a herbal remedy for ailments such as muscle spasms, vomiting, intestinal infections & the common cold.

Cucumber

As well as aiding healthy digestion, cucumbers contain vitamins B1, B5 & B7 which are believed to help ease feelings of anxiety.

Pineapple

As well as being deliciously sweet pineapples contain high amounts of vitamin C and manganese as well as being a good course of dietary fibre and the enzyme bromelain.

Blueberries

Blueberries are now one of the most popular of all eating berries. Coming second only to strawberries in the U.S. they have one of the highest antioxidant capacities among all fruit & vegetables which helps to optimize health by combating the free radicals that can damage cellular structures as well as DNA.

Ginger

The original herbal remedy: amongst many other uses fresh ginger is thought to reduce the symptoms of motion sickness as well as nausea and vomiting associated with morning sickness.

Of course the most common ingredient in any of the recipes is water and the type of water you should use is a hotly contested issue. Broadly speaking tap water is fine but if you can use filtered water you will find it is generally better tasting & smelling as it removes chlorine & bacterial contaminants and balances the pH of the water.

We hope you enjoy our delicious fruit infused water recipes and have fun creating your own!

ALL RECIPES ARE A GUIDE ONLY

All the recipes in this book are a guide only. You may need to alter quantities to suit your own fruit infusing container..

ABOUT COOKNATION

CookNation is the leading publisher of innovative and practical recipe books for the modern, health conscious cook.

CookNation titles bring together delicious, easy and practical recipes with their unique approach - easy and delicious, no-nonsense recipes - making cooking for diets and healthy eating fast, simple and fun.

With a range of #1 best-selling titles - from the innovative 'Skinny' calorie-counted series, to the 5:2 Diet Recipes collection - CookNation recipe books prove that 'Diet' can still mean 'Delicious'!

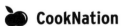 CookNation

Skinny
FRUIT-INFUSED
WATER
RECIPES

GRAPEFRUIT & APPLE WATER

Ingredients

- ½ grapefruit
- ½ apple
- 750ml/3 cups cold water

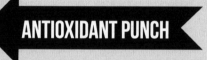

ANTIOXIDANT PUNCH

Method

1 Cut the grapefruit and apple into medium sized slices.

2 Add the fruit to the fruit basket and place inside the water bottle.

3 Top up with as much of the water as you need and close the lid tightly.

4 Leave to infuse in the fridge for an hour or two. Grab your bottle and go.

5 If you want to use a larger fruit infuser pitcher or jug instead of a bottle just double up the quantities and add a handful of ice.

CHEFS NOTE
For extra sweetness try adding a little pineapple to this juice too.

STRAWBERRY & TANGERINE WATER

Ingredients

- Handful of fresh strawberries
- ½ tangerine
- 750ml/3 cups cold water

SUMMER STRAWBERRIES

Method

1 Slice the strawberries.

2 Peel the tangerine and cut each of the segments in half.

3 Add the fruit to the fruit basket and place inside the water bottle.

4 Top up with as much of the water as you need and close the lid tightly.

5 Leave to infuse in the fridge for an hour or two. Grab your bottle and go.

6 If you want to use a larger fruit infuser pitcher or jug instead of a bottle just double up the quantities and add a handful of ice.

CHEFS NOTE
Don't worry about removing the green tops from the strawberries when you slice them up.

CITRUS MINT WATER

Ingredients

- Handful of fresh strawberries
- ¼ orange
- 4-6 fresh mint leaves
- 750ml/3 cups cold water

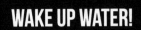

WAKE UP WATER!

Method

1 Slice the strawberries.

2 Peel the orange and cut each of the segments in half.

3 Twist the mint leaves and gently rub in your hands for a moment or two.

4 Add the fruit and mint to the fruit basket and place inside the water bottle.

5 Top up with as much of the water as you need and close the lid tightly.

6 Leave to infuse in the fridge for an hour or two. Grab your bottle and go.

CHEFS NOTE

Twisting and gently rubbing the mint keeps the leaves intact but releases their flavour.

STRAWBERRY LIME SPRITZER

Ingredients

- Handful of fresh strawberries
- ¼ lime
- 750ml/3 cups cold sparkling water

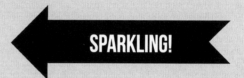

SPARKLING!

Method

1 Slice the strawberries and lime.

2 Add the fruit to the fruit basket and place inside the water bottle.

3 Top up with as much of the sparkling water as you need and close the lid tightly.

4 Leave to infuse in the fridge for half an hour. Grab your bottle and go.

5 If you want to use a larger fruit infuser pitcher or jug instead of a bottle just double up the quantities and add a handful of ice.

CHEFS NOTE
Still water works just fine with this zesty drink too.

LEMON WATER WITH BLUEBERRIES & MINT

Ingredients

- ¼ lemon
- Handful of fresh blueberries
- 4-6 fresh mint leaves
- 750ml/3 cups cold water

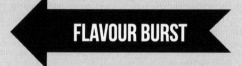

FLAVOUR BURST

Method

1 Using a sharp knife thinly slice the lemon and halve the blueberries.

2 Twist the mint leaves and gently rub in your hands for a moment or two.

3 Add the fruit and mint to the fruit basket and place inside the water bottle.

4 Top up with as much of the water as you need and close the lid tightly.

5 Leave to infuse in the fridge for an hour or two. Grab your bottle and go.

CHEFS NOTE
Frozen blueberries will also work in this simple recipe.

PINEAPPLE BLUEBERRY INFUSED WATER

Makes 1 Fruit Infuser Water Bottle

Ingredients

- 1 thick pineapple ring
- Handful of fresh blueberries
- 750ml/3 cups cold water

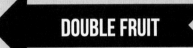

DOUBLE FRUIT

Method

1 Using a sharp knife cut the pineapple into chunks and halve the blueberries.

2 Add the fruit to the fruit basket and place inside the water bottle.

3 Top up with as much of the water as you need and close the lid tightly.

4 Leave to infuse in the fridge for an hour or two. Grab your bottle and go.

CHEFS NOTE
Use fresh or tinned pineapple, either is fine.

LIME CUCUMBER MINT WATER

Ingredients

- ¼-½ lime
- 4cm/2 inch slice of cucumber
- 2-4 fresh mint leaves
- 750ml/3 cups cold water

BRIGHT & FRESH!

Method

1 Using a sharp knife thinly slice the lime and cucumber.

2 Twist the mint leaves and gently rub in your hands for a moment or two.

3 Add the lime, cucumber & mint to the fruit basket and place inside the water bottle.

4 Top up with as much of the water as you need and close the lid tightly.

5 Leave to infuse in the fridge for an hour or two. Grab your bottle and go.

CHEFS NOTE
Reduce the lime if you find it is overpowering the cucumber.

PEACH MINT WATER

Makes 1 Fruit
Infuser Water
Bottle

Ingredients

- 4-6 fresh mint leaves
- ½ - 1 fresh peach
- 750ml/3 cups cold water

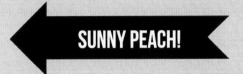

SUNNY PEACH!

Method

1 Slice and cube the peach, discarding the stone.

2 Twist the mint leaves and gently rub in your hands for a moment or two.

3 Add the peach pieces and mint to the fruit basket and place inside the water bottle.

4 Top up with as much of the water as you need and close the lid tightly.

5 Leave to infuse in the fridge for an hour or two. Grab your bottle and go.

CHEFS NOTE

Frozen peace slices are great for using in this recipe to cut down on your prep time.

WATERMELON & ROSEMARY WATER

Makes 1 Fruit Infuser Water Bottle

Ingredients

- 1 watermelon wedge
- 1-2 sprigs of fresh rosemary
- 750ml/3 cups cold water

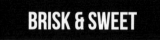 **BRISK & SWEET**

Method

1 Cut the watermelon into chunks.

2 Bash the rosemary with a rolling pin a couple of times to release its flavour.

3 Add the melon and rosemary sprigs to the fruit basket and place inside the water bottle.

4 Top up with as much of the water as you need and close the lid tightly.

5 Leave to infuse in the fridge for an hour or two. Grab your bottle and go.

6 If you want to use a larger fruit infuser pitcher or jug instead of a bottle just double up the quantities and add a handful of ice.

CHEFS NOTE
Quick and easy this fruit water benefits from rosemary's lovely fragrant qualities.

STRAWBERRY, MINT & LEMON WATER

Ingredients

- ¼ lemon
- Handful of strawberries
- 4-6 fresh mint leaves
- 750ml/3 cups cold water

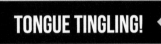

TONGUE TINGLING!

Method

1 Thinly slice the lemon and strawberries.

2 Twist the mint leaves and gently rub in your hands for a moment or two.

3 Add the fruit & mint to the fruit basket and place inside the water bottle.

4 Top up with as much of the water as you need and close the lid tightly.

5 Leave to infuse in the fridge for an hour or two. Grab your bottle and go.

CHEFS NOTE
Mint is a great addition to infused water drinks. It has one of the highest antioxidant capacities of any food.

GINGER ORANGE FRUIT INFUSED WATER

Ingredients

- ½-1 orange
- 2cm/1 inch chunk fresh ginger
- 750ml/3 cups cold water

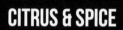

CITRUS & SPICE

Method

1 Peel the orange, break into segments and cut each segment in half.

2 Peel the ginger root and thinly slice.

3 Add the orange and ginger to the fruit basket and place inside the water bottle.

4 Top up with as much of the water as you need and close the lid tightly.

5 Leave to infuse in the fridge for an hour or two. Grab your bottle and go.

6 If you want to use a larger fruit infuser pitcher or jug instead of a bottle just double up the quantities and add a handful of ice.

CHEFS NOTE
Ginger has time-tested health benefits including digestion-friendly properties.

ROSEMARY & STRAWBERRY DETOX WATER

Ingredients

- Handful of fresh strawberries
- 1 sprig of fresh rosemary
- 750ml/3 cups cold water

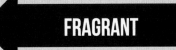

FRAGRANT

Method

1 Slice the strawberries.

2 Bash the rosemary with a rolling pin a couple of times to release its flavour.

3 Add the fruit and rosemary sprig to the fruit basket and place inside the water bottle.

4 Top up with as much of the water as you need and close the lid tightly.

5 Leave to infuse in the fridge for an hour or two. Grab your bottle and go.

6 If you want to use a larger fruit infuser pitcher or jug instead of a bottle just double up the quantities and add a handful of ice.

CHEFS NOTE
Rosemary is often used as a natural remedy to help treat indigestion.

TANGERINE, CUCUMBER & STRAWBERRY WATER

Ingredients

- ½-1 tangerine
- 2 fresh strawberries
- 4cm/2 inch slice of cucumber
- 750ml/3 cups cold water

REFRESHING!

Method

1 Peel the tangerine, break into segments and cut each segment in half.

2 Using a sharp knife thinly slice the strawberries and cucumber.

3 Add the fruit & cucumber to the fruit basket and place inside the water bottle.

4 Top up with as much of the water as you need and close the lid tightly.

5 Leave to infuse in the fridge for an hour or two. Grab your bottle and go.

CHEFS NOTE
This triple combination makes a refreshing morning drink.

PINEAPPLE & ORANGE INFUSED WATER

Ingredients

- ½ orange
- 1-2 thick pineapple rings
- 750ml/3 cups cold water

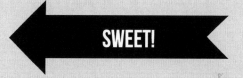

SWEET!

Method

1 Peel the orange, break into segments and cut each segment in half.

2 Chop up the pineapple, add the fruit to the fruit basket and place inside the water bottle.

3 Top up with as much of the water as you need and close the lid tightly.

4 Leave to infuse in the fridge for an hour or two. Grab your bottle and go.

CHEFS NOTE
Double fruit makes this a naturally sweet infused water drink.

SIMPLE APPLE CINNAMON WATER

Ingredients

- ½-1 green apple
- 1 small cinnamon stick
- 750ml/3 cups cold water

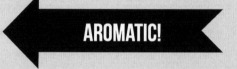

AROMATIC!

Method

1 Core the apple and thinly slice.

2 Add the apple slices and cinnamon stick to the fruit basket and place inside the water bottle.

3 Top up with as much of the water as you need and close the lid tightly.

4 Leave to infuse in the fridge for an hour or two. Grab your bottle and go.

5 If you want to use a larger fruit infuser pitcher or jug instead of a bottle just double up the quantities and add a handful of ice.

CHEFS NOTE
Don't try using ground cinnamon as it will dissolve into the water and won't taste so good.

CHILLED CUCUMBER LEMON WATER

Makes 1 Fruit
Infuser Water
Bottle

Ingredients

- ¼-½ lemon, thinly sliced
- 4cm/2 inch slice of cucumber
- 750ml/3 cups cold water

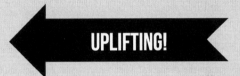
UPLIFTING!

Method

1 Using a sharp knife thinly slice the lemon and cucumber.

2 Add the lemon & cucumber to the fruit basket and place inside the water bottle.

3 Top up with as much of the water as you need and close the lid tightly.

4 Leave to infuse in the fridge for an hour or two. Grab your bottle and go.

CHEFS NOTE
You could add a handful of ice if you want to speed up the chilling process.

HONEYDEW MOJITO WATER

Ingredients

- 1 wedge honeydew melon
- ¼-½ lime
- 4-6 fresh mint leaves
- 750ml/3 cups cold water

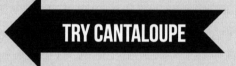

TRY CANTALOUPE

Method

1 Dice the melon and slice the lime.

2 Twist the mint leaves and gently rub in your hands for a moment or two.

3 Add the fruit & mint to the fruit basket and place inside the water bottle.

4 Top up with as much of the water as you need and close the lid tightly.

5 Leave to infuse in the fridge for an hour or two. Grab your bottle and go.

CHEFS NOTE
Use any type of melon you prefer for this simple refreshing drink.

MANGO GINGER WATER

Ingredients

- 2cm/1 inch ginger root
- ½ fresh mango
- 750ml/3 cups cold water

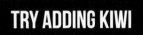
TRY ADDING KIWI

Method

1 Peel the ginger and thinly slice.

2 Peel, de-stone and cube the mango.

3 Add the fruit and sliced ginger to the fruit basket and place inside the water bottle.

4 Top up with as much of the water as you need and close the lid tightly.

5 Leave to infuse in the fridge for an hour or two. Grab your bottle and go.

CHEFS NOTE
It's fine to use frozen mango if that's what you have to hand.

ALLSPICE BERRY & FRUIT INFUSED WATER

Ingredients

- ½-1 tangerine
- 1 tbsp dried cranberries
- ½ tsp whole allspice berries
- 750ml/3 cups cold water

← TRY FRESH CRANBERRIES

Method

1 Peel the tangerine, break into segments and cut each segment in half.

2 Add the fruit and spice berries to the fruit basket and place inside the water bottle. If the allspice berries or cranberries are too small to be held securely in the basket wrap them in a little muslin or other porous cloth.

3 Top up with as much of the water as you need and close the lid tightly.

4 Leave to infuse in the fridge for an hour or two. Grab your bottle and go.

CHEFS NOTE
Allspice berries have a sweet flavour reminiscent of cinnamon, nutmeg & cloves.

COLD PEAR CINNAMON WATER

Ingredients

- ½-1 pear
- 1 cinnamon Stick
- 750ml/3 cups cold water

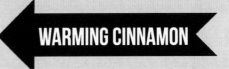

WARMING CINNAMON

Method

1 Core the pear and thinly slice.

2 Snap the cinnamon stick in two.

3 Add the fruit and cinnamon halves to the fruit basket and place inside the water bottle.

4 Top up with as much of the water as you need and close the lid tightly.

5 Leave to infuse in the fridge for an hour or two. Grab your bottle and go.

CHEFS NOTE

Don't use ground cinnamon, only whole cinnamon sticks will do.

MANGO & BASIL WATER

Ingredients

- ½ ripe mango
- 4-6 fresh basil leaves
- 750ml/3 cups cold water

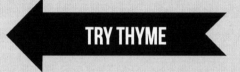 **TRY THYME**

Method

1 Peel, de-stone and cube the mango.

2 Twist the basil leaves and gently rub in your hands for a moment or two.

3 Add the mango and basil leaves to the fruit basket and place inside the water bottle.

4 Top up with as much of the water as you need and close the lid tightly.

5 Leave to infuse in the fridge for an hour or two. Grab your bottle and go.

CHEFS NOTE
Frozen mango will work just fine with this infused water and will speed up the chilling process.

ORANGE GRAPE WATER

Ingredients

- ½ orange
- Handful of seedless grapes
- 750ml/3 cups cold water

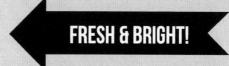

FRESH & BRIGHT!

Method

1 Peel the orange, break into segments and cut each segment in half.

2 Slice the grapes in half.

3 Add the fruit to the fruit basket and place inside the water bottle.

4 Top up with as much of the water as you need and close the lid tightly.

5 Leave to infuse in the fridge for an hour or two. Grab your bottle and go.

CHEFS NOTE
Nutrient dense grapes are particularly good for hydration.

PINK GRAPEFRUIT & ROSEMARY WATER

Ingredients

- ½-1 pink grapefruit
- 1 sprig of fresh rosemary
- 750ml/3 cups cold water

← CONTROLS BLOOD SUGAR

Method

1 Peel the grapefruit, break into segments and cut each segment into quarters.

2 Add the grapefruit and rosemary to the fruit basket and place inside the water bottle.

3 Top up with as much of the water as you need and close the lid tightly.

4 Leave to infuse in the fridge for an hour or two. Grab your bottle and go.

CHEFS NOTE
Leave the rosemary sprig whole but give it a bash with a rolling pin if you want to release more of its flavour into the water.

DOUBLE FRUIT LIME WATER

Ingredients

- Handful of seedless grapes
- ¼ lime
- 2 fresh strawberries
- 750ml/3 cups cold water

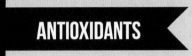
ANTIOXIDANTS

Method

1 Half the grapes and thinly slice the lime & strawberries.

2 Add all the fruit to the fruit basket and place inside the water bottle.

3 Top up with as much of the water as you need and close the lid tightly.

4 Leave to infuse in the fridge for an hour or two. Grab your bottle and go.

CHEFS NOTE
Use a little less lime if you prefer.

SIMPLE MELON WATER

Ingredients

- 1 wedge watermelon
- 750ml/3 cups cold water

CLASSIC!

Method

1 Cube the flesh of the watermelon, discarding the rind.

2 Add the melon to the fruit basket and place inside the water bottle.

3 Top up with as much of the water as you need and close the lid tightly.

4 Leave to infuse in the fridge for an hour or two. Grab your bottle and go.

CHEFS NOTE
The classic combination; it doesn't' get any simpler. When you have finished your drink eat the melon cubes too as a snack.

CHILLED SWEET GREEN TEA

Makes 1 Fruit Infuser Water Bottle

Ingredients

- ½ grapefruit
- ¼ lemon
- 2 tsp maple syrup
- 1 green tea teabag
- 750ml/3 cups cold water

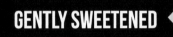
GENTLY SWEETENED

Method

1 Peel the grapefruit, break into segments and cut each segment in half.

2 Using a sharp knife thinly slice the lemon.

3 Drizzle the syrup into the bottom of the water bottle.

4 Add the fruit & teabag to the fruit basket and place inside the water bottle.

5 Top up with as much of the water as you need and close the lid tightly.

6 Check there is no leakage before turning the bottle upside down. Leave to infuse in the fridge (upside down) for an hour or two. Grab your bottle and go.

CHEFS NOTE

Inverting the bottle means the maple syrup should infuse throughout the drink, give it a gently shake if needed.

GRAPE & PINEAPPLE INFUSED WATER

Ingredients

- Handful of seedless red grapes
- 1 thick ring pineapple
- 750ml/3 cups cold water

◄ TRY FROZEN PINEAPPLE

Method

1 Halve the grapes and cube the pineapple.

2 Add all the fruit to the fruit basket and place inside the water bottle.

3 Top up with as much of the water as you need and close the lid tightly.

4 Leave to infuse in the fridge for an hour or two. Grab your bottle and go.

CHEFS NOTE

Pineapple is a source of important vitamins and minerals including thiamin, riboflavin, vitamin B-6, folate, pantothenic acid, magnesium, manganese and potassium.

MANGO MINT INFUSED WATER

Ingredients

- ½ - 1 ripe mango
- 4-6 fresh mint leaves
- 750ml/3 cups cold water

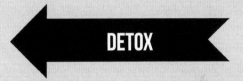

DETOX

Method

1 De-stone the mango, discard the rind and cube the flesh.

2 Twist the mint leaves and gently rub in your hands for a moment or two.

3 Add the mango & mint to the fruit basket and place inside the water bottle.

4 Top up with as much of the water as you need and close the lid tightly.

5 Leave to infuse in the fridge for an hour or two. Grab your bottle and go.

CHEFS NOTE

You can easily refill your bottle with fresh water after drinking, leaving the mango and mint to infuse again for another hour or two.

BASHED RASPBERRIES & MINT WATER

Ingredients

- Handful of fresh raspberries
- 4-6 fresh mint leaves
- 750ml/3 cups cold water

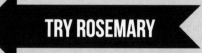

TRY ROSEMARY

Method

1 Twist the mint leaves and gently rub in your hands for a moment or two.

2 Gently crush the raspberries between two spoons, drop straight into the fruit basket and place inside the water bottle along with the mint.

3 Top up with as much of the water as you need and close the lid tightly.

4 Leave to infuse in the fridge for an hour or two. Grab your bottle and go.

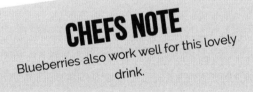

CHEFS NOTE
Blueberries also work well for this lovely drink.

CUCUMBER JALAPEÑO MINT WATER

Makes 1 Fruit Infuser Water Bottle

Ingredients

- 2cm/1 inch slice of cucumber
- ¼ jalapeño pepper
- 2-3 fresh mint leaves
- 750ml/3 cups cold water

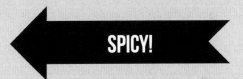

SPICY!

Method

1 Using a sharp knife thinly slice the cucumber.

2 De-seed the jalapeno and slice.

3 Twist the mint leaves and gently rub in your hands for a moment or two.

4 Add the cucumber, jalapeno and mint leaves to the fruit basket and place inside the water bottle.

5 Top up with as much of the water as you need and close the lid tightly.

6 Leave to infuse in the fridge for an hour or two. Grab your bottle and go.

CHEFS NOTE
Adjust the amount of jalapeño pepper to suit your own taste.

MANDARIN, BASIL & BLACK TEA WATER

Ingredients

- ½-1 mandarin orange
- 3-4 basil leaves
- 1 black tea teabag.
- 750ml/3 cups cold water

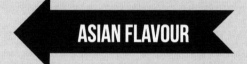

ASIAN FLAVOUR

Method

1 Peel the orange, break into segments and cut each segment in half.

2 Twist the basil leaves and gently rub in your hands for a moment or two.

3 Add the fruit, basil & teabag to the fruit basket and place inside the water bottle.

4 Top up with as much of the water as you need and close the lid tightly.

5 Leave to infuse in the fridge for an hour or two. Grab your bottle and go.

CHEFS NOTE

Widely available, black tea is a type of tea that is generally stronger in flavour than the less oxidized teas.

ORANGE HIBISCUS FLOWER WATER

Ingredients

- ½-1 ripe orange
- 4 hibiscus flowers
- 750ml/3 cups cold water

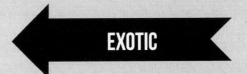

EXOTIC

Method

1 Peel the orange, break into segments and cut each segment in half.

2 Add the orange and flowers to the fruit basket and place inside the water bottle.

3 Top up with as much of the water as you need and close the lid tightly.

4 Leave to infuse in the fridge for an hour or two. Grab your bottle and go.

CHEFS NOTE
This is an exotic combination; you could also try using hibiscus tea instead.

LEMON & CLEMENTINE WATER

Makes 1 Fruit Infuser Water Bottle

Ingredients

- 1 clementine
- ¼ lemon
- 750ml/3 cups cold water

DOUBLE CITRUS

Method

1 Peel the clementine, break into segments and cut each segment in half.

2 Using a sharp knife thinly slice the lemon.

3 Add the fruit to the fruit basket and place inside the water bottle.

4 Top up with as much of the water as you need and close the lid tightly.

5 Leave to infuse in the fridge for an hour or two. Grab your bottle and go.

CHEFS NOTE
Use any type of clementine or tangerine you have to hand.

42

STRAWBERRY LEMON WATER

Makes 1 Fruit Infuser Water Bottle

Ingredients

- Handful of fresh strawberries
- ¼ lemon
- 750ml/3 cups cold water

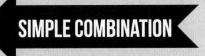

SIMPLE COMBINATION

Method

1 Slice the strawberries and lemon.

2 Add the fruit to the fruit basket and place inside the water bottle.

3 Top up with as much of the water as you need and close the lid tightly.

4 Leave to infuse in the fridge for an hour or two. Grab your bottle and go.

CHEFS NOTE
Make sure the strawberries you use are ripe to get the sweetest flavour.

MIXED HERB INFUSED WATER

Ingredients

- 3-4 leaves fresh basil
- 3-4 leaves fresh mint
- 1 small sprig of rosemary
- 750ml/3 cups cold water

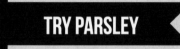 **TRY PARSLEY**

Method

1 Twist the mint & basil leaves and gently rub in your hands for a moment or two.

2 Gently bruise the rosemary sprig with a rolling pin,

3 Add the herbs to the fruit basket and place inside the water bottle.

4 Top up with as much of the water as you need and close the lid tightly.

5 Leave to infuse in the fridge for an hour or two. Grab your bottle and go.

CHEFS NOTE
Use any type of fresh herbs you prefer: thyme and dill add a subtle dimension too.

PINEAPPLE ORANGE WATER

Ingredients

- ½ orange
- 1 thick pineapple slice
- 750ml/3 cups cold water

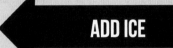

Method

1 Peel the orange, break into segments and cut each segment in half.

2 Cube the pineapple, add the fruit to the fruit basket and place inside the water bottle.

3 Top up with as much of the water as you need and close the lid tightly.

4 Leave to infuse in the fridge for an hour or two. Grab your bottle and go.

CHEFS NOTE
Don't bother peeling the orange if you are short of time, just slice it up.

STRAWBERRY JALAPEÑO INFUSED WATER

Ingredients

- Handful of fresh strawberries
- ¼ jalapeño pepper
- 750ml/3 cups cold water

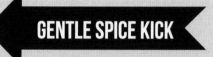

GENTLE SPICE KICK

Method

1 Slice the strawberries, don't worry about discarding the green tops they are fine to leave on.

2 De-seed the jalapeno and slice.

3 Add the strawberries & sliced jalapeno to the fruit basket and place inside the water bottle.

4 Top up with as much of the water as you need and close the lid tightly.

5 Leave to infuse in the fridge for an hour or two. Grab your bottle and go.

CHEFS NOTE
This also works well with fresh raspberries, just slice them in half first.

PINEAPPLE MINT INFUSED WATER

Ingredients

- 4-6 fresh mint leaves
- 1 thick slice fresh pineapple
- 750ml/3 cups cold water

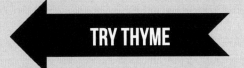

TRY THYME

Method

1 First cube the pineapple.

2 Twist the mint leaves and gently rub in your hands for a moment or two.

3 Add the fruit and mint to the fruit basket and place inside the water bottle.

4 Top up with as much of the water as you need and close the lid tightly.

5 Leave to infuse in the fridge for an hour or two. Grab your bottle and go.

CHEFS NOTE
Tinned pineapple is also fine to use for this recipe too.

RASPBERRY LIME INFUSED WATER

Ingredients

- Small handful of fresh raspberries
- ¼ lime
- 750ml/3 cups cold water

USE RIPE RASPBERRIES

Method

1 Halve the raspberries and thinly slice the lime.

2 Add the fruit to the fruit basket and place inside the water bottle.

3 Top up with as much of the water as you need and close the lid tightly.

4 Leave to infuse in the fridge for an hour or two. Grab your bottle and go.

CHEFS NOTE
Try this with halved fresh cranberries added too.

CUCUMBER MINT DILL WATER

Makes 1 Fruit Infuser Water Bottle

Ingredients

- 4cm/2 inch slice of cucumber
- 1 sprig fresh dill
- 2-3 fresh mint leaves
- 750ml/3 cups cold water

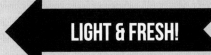

LIGHT & FRESH!

Method

1 Thinly slice the cucumber.

2 Twist the mint leaves and gently rub in your hands for a moment or two.

3 Add the cucumber & herbs to the fruit basket and place inside the water bottle.

4 Top up with as much of the water as you need and close the lid tightly.

5 Leave to infuse in the fridge for an hour or two. Grab your bottle and go.

CHEFS NOTE
Bruise the dill a little before adding to the fruit basket to encourage the flavour to infuse.

WATERMELON & FRESH CORIANDER WATER

Ingredients

- 1 wedge of watermelon
- 4-6 fresh coriander/cilantro leaves
- 750ml/3 cups cold water

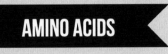

AMINO ACIDS

Method

1 Cube the watermelon flesh, discard the rind.

2 Twist the coriander leaves and gently rub in your hands for a moment or two.

3 Add the melon & coriander to the fruit basket and place inside the water bottle.

4 Top up with as much of the water as you need and close the lid tightly.

5 Leave to infuse in the fridge for an hour or two. Grab your bottle and go.

CHEFS NOTE
The health benefits of coriander include its use in the treatment of skin inflammation and high cholesterol levels.

HONEYDEW SAGE WATER

Makes 1 Fruit
Infuser Water
Bottle

Ingredients

- 1 wedge honeydew melon
- 2-3 fresh sage leaves
- 750ml/3 cups cold water

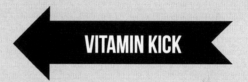

VITAMIN KICK

Method

1 Deseed and cube the melon flesh, discard the rind.

2 Twist the sage leaves and gently rub in your hands for a moment or two.

3 Add the melon and sage to the fruit basket and place inside the water bottle.

4 Top up with as much of the water as you need and close the lid tightly.

5 Leave to infuse in the fridge for an hour or two. Grab your bottle and go.

CHEFS NOTE

Sage has a long history of medicinal use for ailments ranging from mental disorders to gastrointestinal discomfort.

STRAIGHT UP LEMON WATER

Ingredients

- ½-1 lemon
- 750ml/3 cups cold water

QUICK & EASY!

Method

1 Thinly slice the lemon, getting rid of any seeds.

2 Add the lemon slices to the fruit basket and place inside the water bottle.

3 Top up with as much of the water as you need and close the lid tightly.

4 Leave to infuse in the fridge for an hour or two. Grab your bottle and go.

CHEFS NOTE
You will be able to refill and drink this a couple of times without losing the power of the lemon infusion.

PINEAPPLE THYME INFUSED WATER

Makes 1 Fruit
Infuser Water
Bottle

Ingredients

- 1 thick slice fresh pineapple
- 1 sprig fresh thyme
- 750ml/3 cups cold water

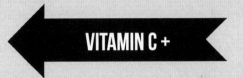

VITAMIN C +

Method

1 First cube the pineapple.

2 Take the sprig of thyme between your palms and gently rub to release the flavour.

3 Add the pineapple and thyme to the fruit basket and place inside the water bottle.

4 Top up with as much of the water as you need and close the lid tightly.

5 Leave to infuse in the fridge for an hour or two. Grab your bottle and go.

CHEFS NOTE

Thyme is an ancient natural remedy. Only recently, however, have researchers pinpointed some of the components in thyme that bring about its healing effects.

STARFRUIT ORANGE WATER

Ingredients

- ½ fresh ripe orange
- 2 thick slices starfruit
- 750ml/3 cups cold water

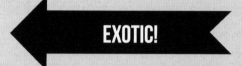

EXOTIC!

Method

1 Peel the orange, break into segments and cut each segment in half.

2 Cube the starfruit slices.

3 Add the fruit to the fruit basket and place inside the water bottle.

4 Top up with as much of the water as you need and close the lid tightly.

5 Leave to infuse in the fridge for an hour or two. Grab your bottle and go.

CHEFS NOTE

Also known as 'carmbola', starfruit used to be an 'exotic' fruit but is now widely available in most large stores.

CHAMOMILE STRAWBERRY & ORANGE WATER

Makes 1 Fruit Infuser Water Bottle

Ingredients

- ¼ ripe fresh orange
- 2 fresh strawberries
- 1 chamomile teabag

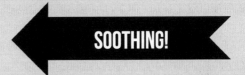

SOOTHING!

Method

1 Cube the orange and slice the strawberries.

2 Add the fruit and teabag to the fruit basket and place inside the water bottle.

3 Top up with as much of the water as you need and close the lid tightly.

4 Leave to infuse in the fridge for an hour or two. Grab your bottle and go.

CHEFS NOTE
Light and refreshing, this is a lovely morning 'pick-me-up'.

LEMON ORANGE BLUEBERRY WATER

Makes 1 Fruit Infuser Water Bottle

Ingredients

- ¼ orange
- ¼ lemon
- Handful of fresh blueberries
- 750ml/3 cups cold water

USE RIPE BLUEBERRIES

Method

1 Peel the orange, break into segments and cut each segment in half.

2 Slice the lemon and halve the blueberries.

3 Add the fruit to the fruit basket and place inside the water bottle.

4 Top up with as much of the water as you need and close the lid tightly.

5 Leave to infuse in the fridge for an hour or two. Grab your bottle and go.

CHEFS NOTE
Try serving this using sparkling water instead.

HERBAL TEA & RASPBERRY WATER

Ingredients

- Handful of fresh raspberries
- 1 herbal teabag
- 750ml/3 cups cold water

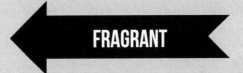

FRAGRANT

Method

1 Slice the raspberries in half.

2 Add the raspberries & teabag to the fruit basket and place inside the water bottle.

3 Top up with as much of the water as you need and close the lid tightly.

4 Leave to infuse in the fridge for an hour or two. Grab your bottle and go.

CHEFS NOTE
Any subtle herbal tea will work well: chamomile or vanilla tea makes a particularly good companion to the fresh raspberries.

LEMONGRASS MINT INFUSED WATER

Makes 1 Fruit Infuser Water Bottle

Ingredients

- 1 lemongrass stalk
- 4-6 fresh mint leaves
- 750ml/3 cups cold water

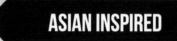

ASIAN INSPIRED

Method

1 Thinly slice the lemongrass stalk lengthways.

2 Twist the mint leaves and gently rub in your hands for a moment or two.

3 Add the lemongrass and mint to the fruit basket and place inside the water bottle.

4 Top up with as much of the water as you need and close the lid tightly.

5 Leave to infuse in the fridge for an hour or two. Grab your bottle and go.

CHEFS NOTE
Lemongrass and mint are a classic Asian combination often used in traditional herbal teas.

SPARKLING ORANGE & BASIL

Makes 1 Fruit Infuser Water Bottle

Ingredients

- ½-1 orange
- 4-6 fresh basil leaves.
- 750ml/3 cups cold sparkling water

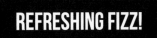

REFRESHING FIZZ!

Method

1 Peel the orange, break into segments and cut each segment in half.

2 Twist the basil leaves and gently rub in your hands for a moment or two.

3 Add the orange & basil to the fruit basket and place inside the water bottle.

4 Top up with as much of the sparkling water as you need and close the lid tightly.

5 Leave to infuse in the fridge for half an hour. Grab your bottle and go.

CHEFS NOTE

Try using lemon thyme instead of basil in this lovely sparkling drink.

LEMON POMEGRANATE INFUSED WATER

Ingredients

- ½-1 pomegranate fruit
- ¼ lemon
- 750ml/3 cups cold water

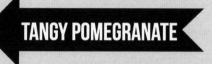
TANGY POMEGRANATE

Method

1 Thinly slice the lemon.

2 Slice the pomegranate thickly, then half the slices leaving the pomegranates seeds still held in the frame of the fruit.

3 Add the to the fruit basket along with the lemon and place inside the water bottle.

4 Top up with as much of the water as you need and close the lid tightly.

5 Leave to infuse in the fridge for an hour or two. Grab your bottle and go.

CHEFS NOTE
If your water bottle can hold very small fruit remove the seeds from the pomegranate and add them along with the lemon into the basket.

BASHED BLACKBERRIES & CITRUS WATER

Ingredients

- Handful of fresh blackberries
- 1 thick slice lime
- 1 thick slice orange.
- 750ml/3 cups cold water

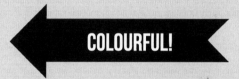

COLOURFUL!

Method

1 Add the lime and orange to the fruit basket.

2 Gently crush the blackberries between two spoons, drop straight into the fruit basket and place inside the water bottle.

3 Top up with as much of the water as you need and close the lid tightly.

4 Leave to infuse in the fridge for an hour or two. Grab your bottle and go.

CHEFS NOTE
The bashed blackberries will turn this water a lovely vibrant colour.

FRESH MINT & PEPPERMINT WATER

Makes 1 Fruit Infuser Water Bottle

Ingredients

- 2-4 fresh mint leaves
- 1 peppermint teabag
- 750ml/3 cups cold water

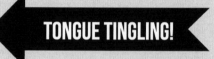 TONGUE TINGLING!

Method

1 Twist the mint leaves and gently rub in your hands for a moment or two.

2 Add the mint leaves and peppermint teabag to the fruit basket and place inside the water bottle.

3 Top up with as much of the water as you need and close the lid tightly.

4 Leave to infuse in the fridge for an hour or two. Grab your bottle and go.

CHEFS NOTE
Fresh lemongrass makes a good addition to this refreshing drink.

CUCUMBER ROSEMARY FENNEL WATER

Makes 1 Fruit Infuser Water Bottle

Ingredients

- 1 fennel top
- 1 sprig rosemary
- 4cm/2 inch slice of cucumber
- 750ml/3 cups cold water

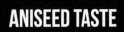
ANISEED TASTE

Method

1 Chop the fennel top and give the rosemary sprig a bash with a rolling pin.

2 Thinly slice the cucumber.

3 Add the fruit, fennel & rosemary to the fruit basket and place inside the water bottle.

4 Top up with as much of the water as you need and close the lid tightly.

5 Leave to infuse in the fridge for an hour or two. Grab your bottle and go.

CHEFS NOTE
The feathery top of the fennel has an aniseed flavour which will add an unusual dimension to your water.

LEMON & GINGER GREEN TEA WATER

Makes 1 Fruit Infuser Water Bottle

Ingredients

- 2cm/1 inch fresh ginger root
- ¼ lemon
- 1 green teabag
- 750ml/3 cups cold water

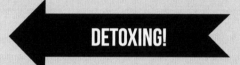

DETOXING!

Method

1 Using a sharp knife peel the ginger and thinly slice along with the lemon.

2 Add the fruit, ginger & teabag to the fruit basket and place inside the water bottle.

3 Top up with as much of the water as you need and close the lid tightly.

4 Leave to infuse in the fridge for an hour or two. Grab your bottle and go.

CHEFS NOTE
The fresh ginger should give this water a warm spicy tingle.

SPARKLING FENNEL WATER

Ingredients

- 2 fennel tops
- 750ml/3 cups cold sparkling water

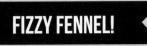

FIZZY FENNEL!

Method

1 Chop the feathery fennel tops and add to the fruit basket.

2 Place inside the water bottle.

3 Top up with as much of the water as you need and close the lid tightly.

4 Leave to infuse in the fridge for an hour or two. Grab your bottle and go.

CHEFS NOTE

There are three main types of fennel; sweet fennel will give you the best result.

LAVENDER AND PEPPERMINT WATER

Ingredients

- Small handful of whole fresh lavender flowers
- 1 peppermint teabag
- 750ml/3 cups cold water

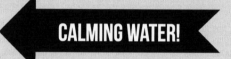

CALMING WATER!

Method

1 Add the lavender and teabag to the fruit basket and place inside the water bottle.

2 Top up with as much of the water as you need and close the lid tightly.

3 Leave to infuse in the fridge for an hour or two. Grab your bottle and go.

CHEFS NOTE
Lavender is believed to have calming and relaxing properties.

![CookNation logo] CookNation

Other
COOKNATION TITLES

If you enjoyed 'The Skinny Fruit-Infused Water Recipe Book' we'd really appreciate your feedback. Reviews help others decide if this is the right book for them so a moment of your time would be appreciated.

Thank you.

You may also be interested in other '**Skinny**' titles in the CookNation series. You can find these and all great titles by searching under '**CookNation**'.

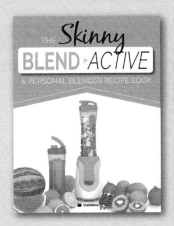

GREAT TASTING, NUTRITIOUS SMOOTHIES, JUICES & SHAKES. PERFECT FOR WORKOUTS, WEIGHT LOSS & FAT BURNING. BLEND & GO!

ISBN 978-1-910771-12-9

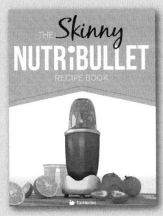

80+ DELICIOUS & NUTRITIOUS HEALTHY SMOOTHIE RECIPES. BURN FAT, LOSE WEIGHT AND FEEL GREAT!

ISBN 978-1-909855-57-1

Printed in Great Britain
by Amazon.co.uk, Ltd.,
Marston Gate.